Straightening the Curve:

The Definitive Approach to Beating Neck Hump

By

Sandra J. Madden

Table of Contents

INTRODUCTION

In a society where looks often affect our perceptions, the human body carries a significant significance. It is our vessel, identity, and medium for contact with the world. In many respects, we are characterized by how we display ourselves. Our posture, gait, and spine alignment play crucial roles in the narrative we compose for ourselves in the physical realm.

In the magnificent tapestry of the human form, the spine is the principal protagonist, functioning as a solid foundation that sustains our existence. But, like with any tale, the spine is not immune to its share of problems, and one of the most prominent challenges is the subject of our exploration: the neck hump.

The neck hump, commonly known as kyphosis or dowager's hump, is a condition that transcends mere aesthetics. It has a dramatic impact on an individual's well-being, both physically and emotionally. It affects posture, impairs movement, and can be a source of discomfort or even pain. But beyond these physical qualities, the neck hump carries a story of resilience, adaptation, and metamorphosis. It is a tale of the body's power to respond to adversity and the journey of individuals who seek to comprehend, address, and finally conquer it.

In this book, we go into the depths of the neck hump, investigating its origins, impact on our lives, and how we can navigate this challenging terrain. Together, we will uncover the subtleties of kyphosis, shedding light on its causes, its repercussions, and the way to a life where the spine stands tall and where the narrative is one of strength, balance, and success.

Join us on this journey of discovery, as we explore the multiple dimensions of the neck hump, and begin on a quest to find the wisdom and empowerment that lay hidden beneath its surface.

CHAPTER ONE

UNDERSTANDING THE NECK HUMP

What Is Neck Hump?

Neck hump, dowager's hump, text hump, hunchback, or round back. The extreme bend of your spine goes by many names. It may grow in either gender, although it derives its name "dowager's hump" from the slightly rounded hunch you could see at the base of an old woman's neck.

This disease, formally termed kyphosis, arises from a chronic, forward-leaning posture that's too prevalent in our world of computer screens and other gadgets. Over time, a tendency of bad posture might cause you to develop an uneven curvature of your upper spine.

Considered a spinal illness, kyphosis is when your spine bends abnormally forward. Your spine has a natural curvature, which helps you stand straight and maintain your posture, but kyphosis may impair your posture and make standing difficult.

Alongside having a hump in your upper back, you may also experience:

- Rounded shoulders.

- Tight hamstrings.
- Pain or stiffness in your back and shoulder blades.
- Extreme tiredness.
- Headaches or migraines

Hyperkyphosis, when the curvature of your spine is excessive, is connected to poor lung function, limited functional ability, and greater mortality.

Often, a dowager's hump is mistaken for a buffalo hump, a condition that has a similar look. A buffalo hump is commonly an indication of Cushing's syndrome. If you have Cushing's disease, you generate extra cortisol, which may lead to excessive fat formation. This extra fat sometimes gathers behind the neck, forming what is commonly referred to as the buffalo hump. Both issues might occur simultaneously or separately.

Types of Neck Hump

There are different forms of neck hump, each with its causes and features. Here are some of the most frequent types:

1. **Postural Neck Hump (Postural Kyphosis):** This is the most typical kind of neck hump and is often associated with poor posture. It occurs from persistent slouching or hunching of the upper back and neck. Postural neck hump may be reversible with better posture and physical treatment.

2. **Age-Related Neck Hump:** As individuals age, the predicted degeneration of spinal discs and bones may lead to an increased curvature of the upper spine. This is commonly found in older persons and may be tied to osteoporosis or other age-related anomalies in the spine.

3. **Scheuermann's Kyphosis:** Scheuermann's disease is a condition that typically affects teenagers and is characterized by the abnormal growth of the vertebrae. It may result in an exaggerated forward curvature of the thoracic spine, resulting in a pronounced neck hump.

4. **Congenital Kyphosis:** Some people are born with defects in the development of their spine, resulting in congenital kyphosis. This form of neck hump is present from birth and may need surgical treatment in extreme circumstances.

5. **Secondary Kyphosis:**** This form of neck hump is caused by underlying medical conditions or events such as:

   - **Osteoporosis:** Weakening of the bones may lead to spinal compression fractures, causing a kyphotic curvature.

   - **Hormonal Imbalances:** Certain hormonal disorders might alter bone health and lead to kyphosis.

   - **Spinal Injuries:** Trauma to the spine, such as fractures or dislocations, may result in a neck hump.

   - **Tumors:** Spinal tumors may cause abnormalities in the curvature of the spine and produce a hump.

6. **Dowager's Hump:** This word is occasionally used informally to refer to an age-related neck hump, particularly in elderly ladies. It may be correlated with osteoporosis-related vertebral fractures.

General Causes of Neck Hump

The creation of a neck hump, known as kyphosis or dowager's hump, might be associated with numerous causes and risk factors. Understanding these features may aid in prevention and treatment. Here are the key reasons and risk factors:

1. **Improper posture:** One of the primary causes of neck hump is bad posture, especially the tendency of slouching or hunch the upper back and neck. Prolonged durations of sitting with rounded shoulders and a forward head position may contribute to the development of kyphosis.
2. **Age:** As individuals age, natural changes occur in the spine, including weakening spinal discs and bones. These age-related changes could raise the incidence of kyphosis, particularly in the thoracic spine (upper back).
3. **Osteoporosis:** Osteoporosis is a disorder characterized by weakened bones, putting patients more prone to fractures. Vertebral compression fractures, prevalent in adults with osteoporosis, may result in an excessive spine curvature and a pronounced neck hump.
4. **Genetics:** There may be an inherited propensity to develop kyphosis in certain conditions. If family members have a

history of spinal curvature diseases, a person may be at a greater risk.

5. **Congenital Factors:** Congenital kyphosis occurs when a person is born with defects in the development of their spine. These defects may lead to an extreme curvature, including a neck hump.

6. **Scheuermann's Disease:** Scheuermann's disease is an ailment that generally affects teenagers and is characterized by abnormal development of the vertebrae. This may result in a substantial kyphotic curvature and a neck hump.

7. **Spinal Injuries:** Traumatic spinal injuries, such as fractures or dislocations, may alter the natural spinal curvature and lead to kyphosis.

8. **Hormonal Imbalances:** Certain hormonal disorders, such as hyperparathyroidism and Cushing's disease, might alter bone health and lead to kyphosis.

9. **Spinal Tumors:** Tumors that grow in or around the spine may lead to alterations in the curvature of the spine and possibly produce a neck hump.

10. **Other Medical illnesses:** Some medical problems, especially neuromuscular disorders like muscular dystrophy, may affect muscle strength and spinal alignment, increasing the likelihood of kyphosis.

11. **Lifestyle Factors:** Sedentary lifestyles, lack of regular exercise, and spending longer hours hunched over

electronic devices or workstations may worsen improper posture and boost the possibility of developing kyphosis.

12.   **Gender:** Women, particularly postmenopausal women, are more prone to osteoporosis-related kyphosis and neck hump owing to hormonal changes that affect bone density.

Importance of Addressing Neck Hump

Addressing a neck hump, also known as a dowager's hump or kyphosis, is crucial for numerous reasons, mostly about physical health, aesthetics, and overall well-being. Here are some important reasons why fixing a neck hump is essential:

1. **Improved Posture:** A neck hump is often related to improper posture, which may lead to several musculoskeletal problems. Addressing the hump may assist improve posture, and lessening the neck, shoulders, and back strain.
2. **Pain Relief:** People with neck humps may experience pain and discomfort in their neck, shoulders, and upper back. Correcting the posture and alignment may improve these symptoms and relieve chronic pain.
3. **Enhanced motion:** Neck humps might restrict neck and shoulder mobility. Treating the hump may expand the range of motion in these regions, making normal chores simpler and more pleasant.

4. **Prevention of Further Progression:** Kyphosis increases over time if left untreated. Early treatment may prevent the hump from becoming more noticeable and severe.
5. **Respiratory Benefits:** Severe neck humps may compress the chest and restrict lung expansion, leading to breathing difficulties. Addressing the hump may aid in improving lung function and overall respiratory health.
6. **Aesthetic Improvement:** Many individuals are self-conscious about the look of a neck hump. Addressing it may improve one's physical appearance and promote self-confidence.
7. **Psychological Well-being:** Chronic pain and poor body image linked with a neck hump may affect mental health. Treating the hump may lead to better psychological well-being and overall quality of life.
8. **Reduced Risk of Complications:** Severe kyphosis may elevate the risk of fractures, pressure sores, and other health concerns. Addressing the hump may decrease these hazards.

Addressing a neck hump frequently includes a variety of approaches, including physical therapy, exercises to strengthen the back and neck muscles, lifestyle alterations to promote appropriate posture, and in rare situations, surgical interventions such as bracing or surgery. It's crucial to chat with a healthcare professional or physical therapist for a correct evaluation and a specialized treatment plan to manage a neck hump effectively. Early intervention is frequently more useful in managing this condition and reducing eventual complications.

CHAPTER TWO

ANATOMY OF THE SPINE

What is the spine?

Your spine, or backbone, is your body's fundamental support system. It links diverse aspects of your bone and muscular system. Your spine permits you to sit, stand, walk, twist, and bend. Back injuries, spinal cord disorders and other linked diseases may damage the spine and generate back pain.

What are the various components of the spine?

A spine in excellent health has three natural bends that generate an S-shape. These curves diffuse shocks to your body while also safeguarding your spine from injury. Many distinct parts make up your spine:

Vertebrae: The spine has 33 stacked vertebrae (small bones) that create the spinal canal. The spinal canal is a tube that shields the spinal cord and nerves, shielding them from harm. Most vertebrae move to allow for a range of mobility. The lowest vertebrae (sacrum and coccyx) are glued together and don't move.

Facet joints: These spinal joints have cartilage (a slippery connective tissue) that enables vertebrae to slide against each other. Facet joints allow you to twist and turn, and they give flexibility and stability. These joints might develop arthritis and create back discomfort or neck pain.

Intervertebral disks: These flat, circular cushions occur between the vertebrae and function as the spine's shock absorbers. Each disk contains a soft, gel-like core (the nucleus pulposus) surrounded by a flexible outer ring (the annulus). Intervertebral disks are under continual pressure. A herniated disk may rupture, causing part of the nucleus' gel material to seep out. Herniated disks (sometimes termed bulging, sliding or ruptured disks) may be painful.

Spinal cord and nerves: The spinal cord is a column of nerves that passes through the spinal canal. The chord spans from the head to the lower back. Thirty-one pairs of nerves grow out via vertebral openings (the neural foramen). These nerves convey signals between the brain and muscles.

Soft tissues: Ligaments link the vertebrae to hold the spine in place. Muscles support the spine and aid you in movement. Tendons link muscles to bone and enable mobility.

What are the spine segments?
The 33 vertebrae make up five different spine segments. Starting from the neck and going toward the buttocks (back end), these components include:

Cervical (neck): The top portion of the spine comprises seven vertebrae (C1 to C7). These neck vertebrae enable you to turn, tilt and nod your head. The cervical spine forms an inward C-shape termed a lordotic curvature.

Thoracic (middle back): The chest or thoracic section of the spine includes 12 vertebrae (T1 to T12). Your ribs join to the thoracic spine. This area of the spine bends out slightly to generate a backward C-shape dubbed the kyphotic curve.

Lumbar (lower back): Five vertebrae (L1 to L5) make up the lowest portion of the spine. Your lumbar spine supports the higher regions of the spine. It links to the pelvis and carries most of your body's weight, as well as the stress of lifting and carrying objects. Many back diseases arise in the lumbar spine. The lumbar spine bends inward to form a C-shaped lordotic curvature.

Sacrum: This triangle-shaped bone joins to the hips. The five sacral vertebrae (S1 to S5) fuse while a baby grows in the uterus, which means they don't move. The sacrum and hip bones create a ring called the pelvic girdle.

Coccyx (tailbone): Four fused vertebrae make up this tiny section of bone found towards the bottom of the spine. Pelvic floor muscles and ligaments link to the coccyx.

How the Neck Hump Develops

The neck hump arises as a consequence of several situations. The key explanation is typically improper posture, when folks repeatedly circle their shoulders, slump over, or keep a forward head position. This leads to greater tension on the upper back and neck. Over time, this chronic stress generates an abnormal curvature in the spine, resulting in the usual look of a neck hump.

Additionally, age-related changes, weakening of the muscles that support the spine, spinal traumas, osteoporosis, and other medical conditions may also contribute to the development of kyphosis. These variables might further worsen the curvature and the hump.

The Role of Posture in Spinal Health

Good posture is one of the simplest and easiest techniques to maintain your spine healthy. While it may need some work and attention, practicing an ideal posture will deliver the right back support. This is particularly vital if you spend time sitting in an office chair or standing throughout the day. Sitting and standing with correct alignment stimulates blood flow, helps keep your nerves and blood vessels healthy, and supports your muscles, ligaments, and tendons. People who acquire a practice of adopting an ideal posture are less likely to have associated back and neck discomfort.

There are numerous functions of optimal posture in supporting spine health. Some of them include;

1. **Alignment and Balance:** Good Posture ensures that the spine is appropriately positioned. The spine has natural curves—cervical (neck), thoracic (upper back), lumbar (lower back), and sacral (pelvic region)—that maintain a balanced posture. Proper posture supports these curves, distributing the body's weight evenly and reducing undue stress on any single area of the spine.

2. **Muscle Support:** Maintaining great posture activates the muscles that support the spine. Strong back and core muscles are crucial for supporting the spine and reducing excessive strain. When you maintain adequate posture, these muscles perform effectively to sustain the spine's natural curvature.

3. **Prevention of Strain and Pain:** Poor Posture, such as slouching or hunching, may lead to unequal pressure on the spine, creating muscular fatigue, tension, and pain. Over time, it may result in persistent pain, particularly in the neck, shoulders, and lower back.

4. **Prevention of Structural Issues:** Consistently maintaining excellent posture helps prevent the development of structural disorders including kyphosis (an excessively forward curvature of the upper back), lordosis (excessive inward curvature of the lower back), and scoliosis

(sideways curvature of the spine). These illnesses may cause discomfort and limit movement.

5. **Respiratory Function:** Proper Posture encourages the chest to expand completely, providing higher lung function and easier breathing. Slouching may compromise lung capacity and lead to lower oxygen intake.

6. **Digestive Health:** Good Posture also helps digestive health. When you sit or stand up straight, the digestive organs have greater room to work properly, perhaps eliminating complications like acid reflux or constipation.

7. **Enhanced Confidence and Well-Being:** Maintaining appropriate posture may also boost confidence and emotional well-being. People who stand and sit tall tend to feel more self-assured and joyful, which may have a ripple influence on overall health.

CHAPTER THREE

SYMPTOMS AND DIAGNOSIS

Common Signs and Symptoms

1. **Visible Hump:** The most recognized indicator of kyphosis is a visible hump or curve in the upper back, often towards the base of the neck. This curvature may vary in magnitude and may be more visible when seen from the side. The protrusion is typically what drives persons to seek medical treatment.

2. **Improper Posture:** Individuals with kyphosis often have improper posture indicated by a forward head position and rounded shoulders. The head and neck may protrude forward, while the upper back appears rounded or drooping. This altered posture might be a physical reflection of the underlying spinal curvature.

3. **Back Pain:** Many patients with kyphosis report pain or distress in the upper back, neck, and shoulders. This discomfort may vary from moderate to severe and may occur for numerous causes, including muscle tension, pressure on the spine, and differing biomechanics attributable to the curvature.

4. **Stiffness:** Stiffness in the neck and upper back is a frequent indicator of kyphosis. The curvature and muscle

imbalances associated with the condition might contribute to reduced flexibility and ease of movement in this region.

5. **Reduced Range of Motion:** Due to the aberrant spinal alignment, patients with kyphosis may have a reduced range of motion in the neck and upper back. This may make it tougher to do ordinary duties and may result in discomfort when conducting activities that need a full range of motion.

6. **Muscle Fatigue:** To compensate for the abnormal curvature, the muscles supporting the vertebrae work harder than usual. This may contribute to muscular fatigue, tension, and discomfort, particularly in the upper back and neck region.

7. **Breathing Difficulties:** Severe kyphosis may compress the thoracic cavity, restricting lung capacity. This compression could result in respiratory issues, particularly during strenuous activity. Individuals may have inadequate or problematic respiration.

8. **Reduced Self-Confidence:** The visible presence of a neck protrusion might impede an individual's self-esteem and self-confidence. It may be emotionally difficult to cope with changes in physical appearance and posture.

9. **Neurological Symptoms:** In more severe situations, kyphosis may induce spinal cord compression. This compression may lead to neurological symptoms such as paralysis, numbness, or sensation in the extremities or legs.

In severe instances, it might even result in the loss of bladder or gastrointestinal control.

When to Seek Medical Attention?

Seeking medical assistance for a neck hump is suggested in the following scenarios; • If you see a visible protrusion in your upper back or a notable alteration in your posture, it's an indication that you should visit a healthcare expert. Early identification and action are critical for confronting the illness effectively.

- If you discover that your neck and upper back have a decreased range of motion, making it tougher to conduct commonplace duties or harming your quality of life. Limited mobility in this region may be connected to kyphosis.
- If you develop chronic respiratory issues, visit a healthcare practitioner soon.
- If you have protracted pain, distress, or rigidity in your neck, upper back, or shoulders, it's crucial to seek medical counsel. These symptoms might be connected with kyphosis and may need examination and treatment.
- In circumstances of severe kyphosis or when there are indicators of spinal cord compression, such as paralysis, numbness, or trembling in the extremities or legs, rapid medical intervention is indicated. Neurological symptoms

might signify a more advanced or hazardous stage of the illness.

- If you have an existing neck protrusion, and you find it becomes more apparent or deteriorating over time, visit a healthcare practitioner. This may signify that the illness is developing and needs attention.
- If you suffer a loss of bowel or bladder control in combination with other symptoms or spinal cord compression, get medical assistance shortly. This might be an indication of substantial spinal cord pressure and needs fast care.
- If you have risk factors for kyphosis, such as osteoporosis, a history of spinal injuries, or certain medical disorders, it's a good idea to have frequent check-ups with your healthcare provider to monitor your spine health.

Self-Diagnostic Tests for Neck Hump

While self-diagnosis is not a replacement for a professional medical examination, there are specific self-assessment techniques you may use to discover indications or risk factors related to a neck protrusion (kyphosis). These self-assessment tools may help you notice possible concerns, but it's vital to visit a healthcare specialist for a comprehensive examination and diagnosis. Here are some self-assessment steps:

1. **Visual Inspection:**
   - Stand in front of a full-length mirror.
   - Observe your Posture from the side and front.
   - Check for any visible hump or aberrant curvature in the upper back or neck.

2. **Posture Check:**
   - Pay attention to your everyday posture, particularly while sitting or standing.
   - Notice whether you incline to stoop, arch your shoulders, or carry your head forward.

3. **Pain and Discomfort:**
   - Evaluate if you experience continuous pain, discomfort, or rigidity in your neck, upper back, or shoulders.

4. **Range of Motion:**
   - Check for any limits in your ability to move your neck and upper back comfortably. Can you readily flex or rotate your neck and shoulders without discomfort or stiffness?

5. **Inhaling and Respiratory Symptoms:**
   - Note if you have problems inhaling, particularly during strenuous exertion. Do you feel constricted or have difficulty breathing?

6. **Neurological Symptoms:**
  - Be wary of any signs of neurological symptoms, such as paralysis, numbness, or tingling in your arms or legs.

7. **Risk Factors:**
  - Consider if you have any risk factors for kyphosis, such as a history of spinal injuries, osteoporosis, or certain medical diseases.

CHAPTER FOUR

SPECIFIC TYPES OF KYPHOSIS AND THEIR CAUSES

Postural Kyphosis

Postural kyphosis, also known as postural roundback, is a form of kyphosis that is not commonly correlated with anatomical concerns in the spine. Instead, it is primarily connected to incorrect posture and actions. The causes of postural kyphosis include:

1. **Poor Posture:** The most prominent cause of postural kyphosis is bad posture, particularly in the upper back and neck. Prolonged periods of slouching, hunching, or sustaining a forward head posture may contribute to an excessive curvature of the upper vertebrae.

2. **Habitual Positions:** Spending extensive periods seated or standing with improper spinal alignment, such as while using electronic devices, studying, or working at a desk, may contribute to the development of postural kyphosis.

3. **Muscle Imbalances:** Weakness in the muscles that sustain an erect posture could result in postural kyphosis. When

these muscles are underdeveloped or misused, they are less efficient in sustaining appropriate spinal alignment.

4. **Lack of Physical Activity:** A sedentary lifestyle and a lack of regular exercise may lead to muscle weakness and contribute to postural kyphosis.

5. **Carrying Heavy Backpacks:** Carrying heavy backpacks or luggage on one shoulder may induce postural kyphosis, since it can contribute to unequal pressure on the spine and shoulders.

6. **Habitual repeated movements:** Engaging in repeated actions or postures that stimulate the curvature of the upper spine and neck may lead to postural kyphosis over time.

7. **Ergonomics:** Improper ergonomics in work or study conditions may contribute to improper posture and postural kyphosis. Inadequate desk and chair arrangement, incorrect screen height, and inadequate workstation design may all play a role.

8. **Lack of Awareness:** Many individuals are oblivious to their posture and its influence on their spinal health. Ignoring the requirement of retaining appropriate posture could contribute to the development of postural kyphosis.

9. **Psychosocial Factors:** Stress, anxiety, and emotional factors may also alter posture. Individuals under duress may exhibit rigid, stooped postures, leading to postural kyphosis.

Secondary Kyphosis

Secondary kyphosis is a type of kyphosis that develops as a consequence of an underlying cause or disease. It is vital to identify and address the underlying cause to adequately manage or treat secondary kyphosis. Here are some typical causes:

1. **Osteoporosis:** Osteoporosis is a condition characterized by compromised bones, placing patients more prone to fractures. Vertebral compression fractures are frequent in individuals with osteoporosis, leading to a collapse of one or more vertebrae and the development of kyphosis.
2. **Spinal Injuries:** Traumatic injuries to the spine, such as fractures, dislocations, or spinal cord injuries, may result in abnormalities in spinal alignment and the development of kyphosis.
3. **Connective Tissue Disorders:** Some connective tissue disorders, such as Marfan syndrome and Ehlers-Danlos syndrome, may impair the strength and integrity of the spinal ligaments and connective tissues, resulting in kyphosis.
4. **Neuromuscular Disorders:** Certain neuromuscular illnesses, including muscular dystrophy, may lead to muscle weakness and spinal anomalies, such as kyphosis.
5. **Spinal Tumors:** Tumors that grow in or around the spine may displace and harm the vertebrae, producing kyphosis.

6. **Scheuermann's Disease:** This is a condition that generally affects adolescents and is characterized by the abnormal development of the vertebrae, resulting in an excessive curvature of the spine and kyphosis.
7. **Hormonal Imbalances:** Conditions like hyperparathyroidism and Cushing's disease may impact bone density and lead to kyphosis.
8. **Congenital Factors:** Some individuals are born with congenital defects in the formation of their spine, leading to the development of kyphosis.
9. **Inflammatory illnesses:** Inflammatory illnesses, such as ankylosing spondylitis, may induce inflammation and fusion of the spinal joints, resulting in kyphosis.
10. **Long-Term Poor Posture:** Chronic poor Posture, such as slouching or maintaining a forward head posture, may contribute to muscle imbalances and structural abnormalities in the spine, ultimately terminating in kyphosis.

Age-Related Kyphosis

Age-related kyphosis, frequently referred to as "hyperkyphosis" or "hyperkyphoscoliosis of the spine," is characterized by an excessive forward curvature of the upper spine, resulting in a rounded or bowed back. This condition is often related to the natural aging process and arises for several reasons:

1. **Degenerative Changes:** Over time, the intervertebral discs of the spine progressively degrade. They lose water content and become less robust, resulting in a decline in disc height. As a consequence, the spine's ability to preserve its natural alignment and curvature diminishes.

2. **Osteoporosis:** Osteoporosis is a prevalent age-related condition characterized by a decline in bone density and strength. As bone density diminishes, the vertebrae become more prone to compression fractures. Vertebral compression fractures may contribute to a pronounced forward curvature of the spine, notably in the upper back.

3. **Muscle Weakness:** Aging may result in muscle weakening and a loss in muscle mass, particularly the muscles that support the spine. Weak back and abdominal muscles may make it tougher to maintain an erect posture and sustain the strain of gravity on the vertebrae.

4. **Ligament Stiffness:** The ligaments that hold the vertebrae together could become less flexible with age. This rigidity may limit the spine's ability to maintain optimal alignment.

5. **Joint Changes:** Changes in the facet joints that link the vertebrae may develop with age, possibly altering the spine's curvature.

6. **Gender and Hormonal Factors:** Age-related kyphosis is more likely in women, particularly postmenopausal women. Hormonal changes, notably a reduction in

estrogen, could impact bone health and contribute to kyphosis.

7. **Compression Fractures:** Vertebral compression fractures may occur more often in aged persons because of decreasing bone density, particularly in conjunction with osteoporosis. These fractures could contribute to an excessive forward curvature of the upper vertebrae.

8. **Sedentary Lifestyle:** A lack of physical exercise, particularly weight-bearing activities, may contribute to muscle atrophy and an increased risk of developing age-related kyphosis.

9. **Hereditary Predisposition:** Some individuals may have a hereditary predisposition that renders them more vulnerable to age-related spine changes and curvature.

Congenital Kyphosis

Congenital kyphosis is a kind of kyphosis that is present from birth and is primarily caused by defects in the construction and development of the spine. Several factors may lead to congenital kyphosis:

1. **Vertebral Malformation:** Congenital kyphosis frequently occurs from the abnormal development of one or more vertebral bones in the spine. This may entail malformations such as wedged vertebrae (wedge-shaped bones) or fused vertebrae (two or more vertebrae united).

These abnormalities impact the natural alignment of the spine and result in an unnatural curvature.

2. **Hemivertebrae:** Hemivertebrae are imperfect or imperfectly formed vertebral bodies. They may lead to congenital kyphosis when they are not appropriately aligned with the contiguous vertebrae, causing a wedge-shaped deformity.

3. **Butterfly Vertebrae:** In certain circumstances, congenital kyphosis may be related to butterfly vertebrae, which occur when the vertebral body has a split or divide in the middle, approximating a butterfly shape. This abnormality may contribute to kyphotic curvatures.

4. **Failure of Segmentation:** The spine develops from a sequence of segments in the embryo. Failure of correct segmentation during development may lead to variably developed vertebrae and result in kyphotic curvatures.

5. **Neural Tube Defects:** Conditions like spina bifida, which include partial closure of the neural tube during embryonic development, may be linked with congenital spinal abnormalities, including kyphosis.

6. **Genetic Factors:** There may be a genetic component to congenital kyphosis, since it may run in families. Certain genetic disorders or situations may enhance the possibility of aberrant spine development.

7. **Environmental Factors:** While less frequent, exposure to certain environmental factors during pregnancy may

elevate the prevalence of congenital kyphosis. These factors might include maternal smoking, alcohol consumption, or exposure to specific contaminants.

Scheuermann's Kyphosis

Scheuermann's kyphosis, usually known as Scheuermann's disease, is a malady characterized by an excessive and unnatural forward curvature of the thoracic or thoracolumbar spine. The particular etiology of Scheuermann's kyphosis is not completely known, however, it is believed to originate from a combination of inherited and environmental reasons. Here are some of the likely causes and contributing factors:

1. **Genetics:** There is evidence to infer a genetic component in the development of Scheuermann's kyphosis. It typically runs in families, and those with a family history of the illness may be at a greater risk. Specific genetic characteristics liable for Scheuermann's illness are currently being researched.

2. **Abnormal Growth Plate Development:** Scheuermann's kyphosis is considered to be related to alterations in the growth plates of the vertebral bodies. These growth plates, which are positioned near the extremities of long bones, are responsible for bone development throughout infancy and adolescence. In Scheuermann's illness, the growth plates in the thoracic or thoracolumbar spine may develop

inappropriately, resulting in wedge-shaped vertebrae and excessive forward flexion.

3. **Hormonal Factors:** Hormonal imbalances or anomalies in growth hormone secretion during the adolescent growth phase have been theorized as contributing factors to the development of Scheuermann's kyphosis. These hormonal variations may disrupt the growth plates and spinal development.

4. **Biomechanical Factors:** The mechanical stresses and pressures placed on the spine throughout growth and adolescence might influence the development of Scheuermann's kyphosis. Activities that demand repeated or severe tension on the vertebrae, such as weightlifting or certain sports, may be contributing causes.

5. **Dietary Factors:** In uncommon instances, dietary inadequacies during adolescence have been postulated as potential factors to Scheuermann's kyphosis. Adequate nutrition, including the ingestion of essential vitamins and minerals, is necessary for appropriate bone growth and development.

6. **Environmental conditions:** Certain environmental conditions, such as improper posture, enormous luggage, or job circumstances that entail hard lifting or persistent spinal stress, might potentially exacerbate the disease in those who are genetically prone to it.

CHAPTER FIVE

CONSERVATIVE TREATMENT OPTIONS

Physical Therapy and Exercises

Physical therapy and specialized exercises may be effective for improving posture and decreasing the appearance of a neck hump (kyphosis). These exercises try to strengthen the muscles that support the spine, enhance flexibility, and encourage better posture. However, it's crucial to contact a healthcare specialist or a physical therapist before beginning any fitness program, particularly if you have an existing neck hump or associated spinal difficulties. They may give help customized to your scenario. Here are some general exercises and self-physical therapy techniques:

1. **Chin Tucks:**
   - Sit or stand with your back straight.
   - Gently tuck your chin into your chest.
   - Hold for a few seconds, then release.
   - Repeat this technique to strengthen the neck and upper back muscles and improve head alignment.
2. **Wall Angels:**
   - Stand with your back against a wall.

- Raise your arms, retaining your elbows and wrists in contact with the wall.
- Slowly drop your arms to your sides.
- This exercise helps improve shoulder mobility and upper back posture.

3. Thoracic Extension Stretch:

- Sit or stand with your back straight.
- Interlace your fingers behind your head.
- Gently arch your upper back and elevate your chest.
- Hold for a few seconds, then return to the starting position.
- This stretch helps offset forward head posture and encourages a more upright upper back.

4. Scapular Squeezes:

- Sit or stand with your back straight.
- Squeeze your shoulder blades together.
- Hold for a few seconds, then release.
- This exercise strengthens the muscles between the shoulder blades and gives improved upper back posture.

5. Prone Cobra:

- Lie face down with your arms at your sides.
- Lift your head, chest, and arms off the ground while pressing your shoulder blades together.
- Hold for a few seconds, then lower yourself.

- This exercise improves the muscles of the upper back and neck.

6. **Stretching the Chest Muscles:**
   - Stand in a doorway with your elbows bent at a 90-degree angle.
   - Place your forearms and hands on the doorframe.
   - Step forward with one foot to gently stretch your chest and shoulders.
   - Hold the stretch for 20-30 seconds.
   - This helps to alleviate tightness in the chest, which may lead to improper posture.
- Pilates: Participating in pilates lessons with an emphasis on spinal flexibility, posture, and core strength might be effective for persons with kyphosis.

Consistency is important while doing these exercises. Perform them regularly, but avoid overexertion. It's crucial to maintain proper form and gradually increase the intensity and duration as you gain more experience with the exercises. If you feel any pain or discomfort while executing these exercises, stop immediately and seek a healthcare specialist. They may give individual coaching and verify that the routines are suitable for your condition.

Lifestyle Changes and Ergonomics

Lifestyle adjustments and ergonomic improvements may be useful for controlling and preventing a neck hump (kyphosis).

These adjustments try to improve posture, strengthen supporting muscles, and ease stress on the spine. Here are some practical steps to consider:

1. **Maintain Good Posture:**

- Be attentive to your posture when sitting, standing, and walking. Keep your back straight, shoulders relaxed, and head aligned with your spine.
- Consider utilizing a mirror or posture-correcting equipment to assist in maintaining ideal posture.

2. **Stretching and Strengthening Exercises:**

- Incorporate stretching and strengthening exercises into your daily routine to boost the flexibility and strength of your back and neck muscles. Focus on exercises that target the upper back and neck.
- Consult a physical therapist or fitness trainer for a customized training routine.

3. **Ergonomic workstation:**

- If you work at a desk or computer, ensure that your environment is ergonomically structured. Adjust your chair, monitor, and keyboard to maintain a neutral posture.
- Take frequent pauses to get up, stretch, and move about to reduce lengthy sitting.

4. **Backpack and Bag Usage:**
   - When carrying a backpack or bag, distribute the weight equally on both shoulders. Use backpacks with padded straps and a waist belt for improved weight distribution.
   - Avoid carrying huge weights with one hand or over one shoulder.
5. **Pillow and Mattress Selection:**
   - Choose a supportive pillow and mattress to ensure healthy spinal alignment during sleeping. Your pillow should support your neck, and your mattress should supply ample back support.
6. **Limit Screen Time:**
   - Reduce the time spent gazing down at electronic devices like smartphones or tablets. Hold gadgets at eye level to prevent straining your neck.
7. **Regular Physical exercise:**
   - Engage in regular physical exercise to develop your core and back muscles. Activities such as swimming, yoga, and Pilates may be especially good for posture and spinal health.
8. **Avoid Excessive Lifting:**
   - When lifting bulky products, utilize correct lifting methods. Bend at your knees and keep your back straight to reduce strain on the spine.

9. **Posture Brace:**

- Consider applying a posture brace or support device, particularly if you have trouble sustaining fantastic posture. These gadgets could give reminders to sit or stand upright.

10. **Regular Check-Ups:**

- Schedule regular check-ups with a healthcare practitioner to monitor your spinal health, particularly if you have risk factors for kyphosis.

11. **Avoid Sedentary Behavior:**

- Limit lengthy periods of sitting or inactivity. Stand, walk, and move around at regular intervals to prevent muscle stiffness and spinal tension.

12. **Consult a Specialist:**

- If you have concerns about your posture or suspect you have a neck hump, consult a healthcare professional, orthopedic specialist, or physical therapist for a comprehensive assessment and guidance on personalized strategies for improving your posture and managing the condition.

Lifestyle modifications and ergonomic adjustments may play a substantial role in preventing and managing a neck hump, especially when supported by expert guidance and exercises designed to target the troublesome regions.

Bracing Techniques

Bracing treatments are frequently not the main therapy for a neck hump (kyphosis), since they are more often applied for treating scoliosis, which is a lateral curvature of the spine. Kyphosis is characterized by an excessive forward curvature of the spine in the thoracic or thoracolumbar region. However, in rare instances, particularly when kyphosis is still in the early stages and the spine is flexible, a brace may be employed. Bracing is most often utilized in teens with Scheuermann's kyphosis, which is a particular sort of kyphosis.

Here's a general discussion of bracing techniques for kyphosis:

1. **Type of Brace:** A brace used for kyphosis is frequently a custom-fitted orthosis used to assist in supporting and straightening the spine. One popular form of brace is the Milwaukee brace, which has a neck ring combined with a body garment. Other sorts of braces may also be applied depending on the unique needs of the person.
2. **Patient assessment:** The decision to wear a brace is based on a full assessment by an orthopedic expert. This examination comprises the degree of the kyphosis, flexibility of the spine, the patient's age, and general health. Bracing is routinely examined for teens with mild kyphosis which is still flexible and may improve with bracing.
3. **Brace Wearing:** If a brace is prescribed, the patient is educated on how to wear it. Bracing for kyphosis

frequently necessitates wearing the brace for a predetermined amount of hours each day. The brace delivers external support to the spine and helps to minimize or halt the development of the curvature.

4. **Monitoring and modifications:** Regular follow-up sessions are essential to monitor the efficacy of the brace and make any necessary alterations. The brace may need to be altered as the patient's spine changes.

5. **Physical Therapy:** Often, patients assigned a brace for kyphosis may also engage with a physical therapist to improve posture, strengthen muscles, and learn exercises to complement the therapy.

It's crucial to note that bracing is typically advised for teenagers with flexible kyphosis and is less useful for adults with firm, established curvatures. The ultimate purpose of bracing is to prevent further progression of the kyphosis and induce proper alignment of the spine. In cases where kyphosis is more severe or inflexible, or when other therapies like surgery are essential, bracing may not be the main or only therapeutic choice. The use of a brace should always be discussed with and managed by a trained orthopedic specialist.

CHAPTER SIX

MEDICATIONS AND NON-SURGICAL INTERVENTIONS

Medications for Osteoporosis-Related Kyphosis

Osteoporosis-related kyphosis, which occurs from the weakening and compression of vertebrae owing to inadequate bone density, is generally managed with a combination of therapies to address the underlying osteoporosis and its impact on the spine. Medications are a crucial component of osteoporosis treatment. While medications themselves do not directly cure kyphosis, they strive to boost bone density and minimize the risk of further fractures and deformities. Here are some common medicines used in the therapy of osteoporosis-related kyphosis:

1. **Bisphosphonates:** Bisphosphonates are a family of medications that aid in improving bone density and minimize the risk of fractures. Commonly prescribed bisphosphonates include Alendronate (Fosamax), Risedronate (Actonel), Ibandronate (Boniva), and Zoledronic acid (Reclast). These medications slow the speed of bone loss and boost bone strength.

2. **Selective Estrogen Receptor Modulators (SERMs):** Medications like Raloxifene (Evista) function similarly to

estrogen in select regions of the body and may help prevent bone loss. They are commonly given to postmenopausal women at risk of osteoporosis.

3. **Parathyroid Hormone (Teriparatide):** Teriparatide (Forteo) is a medication that stimulates bone development. It is routinely prescribed for people with severe osteoporosis who are at high risk of fractures.

4. **Calcium and Vitamin D Supplements:** Adequate calcium and vitamin D consumption is necessary for maintaining bone health. Supplements may be recommended to ensure that the body obtains adequate levels of these nutrients.

5. **Monoclonal Antibodies:** Denosumab (Prolia) is a monoclonal antibody that may be injected to treat osteoporosis. It reduces the activity of cells responsible for bone breakdown.

6. **Hormone Replacement Therapy (HRT):** In certain instances, hormone replacement therapy may be suggested, especially for postmenopausal women. Estrogen medicine may help boost bone density, but its usage is carefully examined owing to possible bad effects.

7. **Strontium Ranelate:** Strontium ranelate (Protelos) is a medication that may enhance bone density and lessen the risk of fractures. It's employed in certain locations, however, its usage may be regulated owing to fears about possible bad consequences.

It's vital to stress that the choice of medicine and the treatment plan should be developed by a healthcare expert based on an individual's particular condition, risk factors, and medical history. In the situation of kyphosis, these medications strive to prevent future fractures and spinal compression, which may contribute to the development of kyphosis. Additionally, lifestyle modifications, such as weight-bearing exercises, a balanced diet, and fall prevention strategies, are critical components of osteoporosis management to minimize the risk of future fractures and the development of kyphosis.

Chiropractic Treatment and Alternative Therapies

Chiropractic treatments and alternative therapies might be investigated for relieving a neck hump (kyphosis) as complementary options to standard medical therapy. It's vital to note that the efficacy of different therapies may vary depending on the genesis and severity of the issue. Here's an explanation of how chiropractic treatment and alternative therapies could be utilized:

1. **Chiropractic Care:**
   - **Spinal Adjustment:** Chiropractors may perform manual spinal adjustments to treat misalignments in the spine. While spinal adjustments are a standard chiropractic approach, their efficacy in treating kyphosis may be restricted, especially in individuals with structural abnormalities in the spine.

- **Postural Education:** Chiropractors may give guidance on improving posture. They may give exercises and stretches to develop back and core muscles, which may assist in promoting optimal spinal alignment.
- **Pain Management:** Chiropractic treatment may be beneficial for managing pain and suffering associated with kyphosis. Chiropractors may utilize therapies such as massage, electrical stimulation, or ultrasound therapy to ease the pain.

2. **Physical Therapy:**
- Physical therapists may develop particular exercise routines targeted at improving posture and strengthening the muscles that support the spine. These exercises may help avoid the growth of kyphosis and minimize accompanying pain.

3. **Yoga and Pilates:**
- These mind-body activities may help improve posture, flexibility, and core strength. Regular participation in yoga or Pilates sessions may lead to improved spinal alignment and less kyphosis-related pain.

4. **Massage therapy:**
- Massage treatment may aid in lowering muscular tension and pain associated with kyphosis. While it may not cure the spinal curvature itself, it may give symptomatic relief.

5. Acupuncture:

- Acupuncture may be used to treat pain and muscular tension associated with kyphosis. It's claimed to induce relaxation, reduce pain, and boost overall well-being.

6. Orthopedic Bracing:

- Bracing is a more conventional therapy that may be investigated for teens with kyphosis. An orthopedic brace may aid in supporting the spine and encouraging healthy alignment, especially if the kyphosis is found early.

7. Ergonomic Adjustments:

- Making ergonomic modifications to your employment or home environment could encourage improved posture. This may include optimal workplace and chair ergonomics, utilizing supporting cushions and avoiding extended sitting or standing.

It's vital to visit a healthcare provider before contemplating chiropractic therapy or other cures for kyphosis. They may analyze the source and severity of the condition and propose the most suitable treatment solutions. In certain instances, a combination of medical treatment, physical therapy, and alternative treatments may offer the best complete approach to managing kyphosis and concomitant symptoms.

Pain Management Strategies

Pain therapy for a neck hump, or kyphosis, typically includes several techniques to lessen pain and promote quality of life. It's crucial to consult a healthcare expert for a precise treatment plan, since the approach may change depending on the severity of the condition and the underlying reasons. Here are some pain management strategies:

1. Physical therapy may help improve posture and strengthen the muscles that support the spine. Therapists may give exercises and stretches to reduce pain and stiffness and encourage greater spinal alignment.
2. Over-the-counter pain drugs, such as ibuprofen or acetaminophen, may be used to manage moderate to severe discomfort. In rare cases, prescription medicines may be advised for more severe pain.
3. Applying heat or cold packs to the afflicted regions could help alleviate pain and relax tight muscles. Heat is typically utilized for muscle relaxation, while cold may decrease inflammation and numb the region
4. Learning and maintaining optimal posture may help reduce discomfort by decreasing pressure on the spine. Using ergonomic equipment, such as supportive chairs and pillows, may be advantageous.
5. In rare instances, a brace or orthosis may be administered to help improve posture and reduce discomfort. Bracing is

more often done for teenagers with kyphosis who are still developing.

6. Techniques like chiropractic adjustments or osteopathic manipulation may be utilized to relieve pain and improve spinal alignment.

7. Specific exercises and stretches may help enhance the flexibility of the spine and strengthen the surrounding muscles. • A physical therapist or healthcare practitioner may suggest suitable workouts specific to the individual's condition.

8. In severe situations of significant pain, your healthcare provider may administer epidural injections or nerve blocks to decrease inflammation and relieve discomfort.

9. Lifestyle modifications, particularly weight management, may help lower the pressure on the spine and minimize discomfort.

10. In situations of severe kyphosis or when conservative treatment is ineffective, surgery may be considered. Surgical options include spinal fusion and correction of the curvature. • Relaxation practices, such as deep breathing, mindfulness, or meditation, may help manage pain by lowering stress and tension.

It's vital to see a healthcare practitioner to help pick the most efficient pain management approach depending on your unique condition and demands. A complete assessment will aid find the underlying causes of the neck hump and lead to the design of a suitable treatment approach.

CHAPTER SEVEN

PREVENTING NECK HUMP

Posture Improvement Strategies

Improving your posture is crucial for curing and avoiding a neck hump (kyphosis). Here are some practical techniques to assist you in maintaining a better posture:

1. **Awareness:** The first step in improving posture is being aware of your present posture. Regularly check in with your posture, both while sitting and standing. Use mirrors or even smartphone applications to help you check your alignment.

2. **Ergonomic Workstation:** If you have a desk job, ensure your workstation is ergonomically structured. Use an adjustable chair that supports the natural curvature of your spine. Position your computer display at eye level to avoid bending your head forward.

3. **Frequent pauses:** If you sit for lengthy periods, take frequent intervals to stand, stretch, and move about. Set reminders to prevent extended durations of poor posture.

4. **Strengthen Core and Back Muscles:** Strong core and back muscles are crucial for sustaining healthy posture. Incorporate exercises like planks, bridges, and rows into your workout routine to enhance these muscle groups.

5. **Stretching:** Regularly stretch the muscles that may become stiff due to incorrect posture. Focus on the chest, shoulders, and neck. Simple stretches like the doorway stretch or neck tilts may help reduce stress.

6. **Yoga and Pilates:** These activities may be effective for improving posture and core strength. Consider taking courses or watching instructional videos.

7. **Posture-Correcting gadgets:** Some wearable gadgets and smartphone applications may give real-time feedback on your posture and aid you in making critical improvements.

8. **Physical Therapy:** A physical therapist may give exercises and therapy specific to your posture concerns and help you build healthier habits.

9. **Orthopedic Supports:** If indicated by a healthcare specialist, consider utilizing orthopedic supports like a posture-correcting brace to aid in retraining your muscles and preserving appropriate alignment.

10. **Mindfulness and Mind-Body practices:** Mindfulness practices, such as meditation and tai chi, may help you become more aware of your body and encourage better posture.

11. **Pillow and Mattress Selection:** Ensure your pillow and mattress give proper support for your neck and back. Choose options that adjust your spine while you sleep.

12. **Proper Lifting Techniques:** When lifting heavy things, use your legs, not your back, to reduce pressure on your spine.

13. **Reduce Backpack Weight:** If you use a backpack, make it as light as possible and utilize both shoulder straps to distribute the weight equally.

14. **Self-Monitoring:** Use smartphone apps or wearable devices to monitor your posture and get reminders or alerts when you slouch or maintain bad posture.

15. **Speak with a Healthcare Professional:** If you have an existing neck hump or severe kyphosis, speak with a healthcare professional, such as a physical therapist or orthopedic specialist, for personalized counseling and treatment.

Consistency and patience are necessary since restoring posture is an ongoing process. By adopting these methods and making a deliberate effort to maintain good posture, you may help prevent and reduce a neck hump and minimize the risk of future spine-related diseases.

Exercises for a Healthy Spine

1. **Cat-Cow Stretch:**
   - Start on your hands and knees with a neutral spine.
   - Inhale, arch your back and elevate your head (Cow Pose).

- Exhale, round your back, and tuck your chin (Cat Pose).
- Repeat the process numerous times to warm up the spine.

2. Child's Pose:

- Kneel on the floor with your big toes together and knees apart.
- Sit back on your heels, extend your arms forward, and drop your chest toward the floor.
- This posture stretches and relieves stress in the spine.

3. Cobra Pose:

- Lie face down with your hands beneath your shoulders.
- Inhale and raise your chest off the ground, retaining your hips on the floor.
- This strengthens the lower back and increases flexibility in the spine.

4. Superman Exercise:

- Lie face down with your arms raised above.
- Lift your arms, chest, and legs off the ground simultaneously.
- Hold for a few seconds and then drop.
- This exercise targets the muscles supporting the spine.

5. **Bridges:**
   - Lie on your back with your knees bent and feet flat on the floor.
   - Lift your hips off the ground, working your glutes and core.
   - Lower your hips and repeat.
   - Bridges aid in strengthening the lower back and core muscles.

6. **Planks:**
   - Start in a push-up posture with your elbows on the ground and your body in a straight line.
   - Hold this posture for as long as you can while engaging your core.
   - Planks are wonderful for strengthening the core, which supports the spine.

7. **Side Planks:**
   - Lie on your side with your elbow under your shoulder.
   - Lift your hips off the ground, forming a straight line from head to heels.
   - Perform on both sides to improve the lateral core muscles.

8. **Seated Spinal Twist:**
   - Sit with your legs extended.
   - Bend one knee and put the foot on the outside of the opposite thigh.

- Twist your body and gaze over your shoulder.
- This exercise promotes spinal mobility and flexibility.

9. **Wall Angels:**
- Stand with your back against a wall and arms spread out to the sides.
- Slowly glide your arms up and down the wall while retaining contact.
- Wall Angels enhance shoulder and thoracic spine mobility.

10. **Neck Stretches:**
- Gently tilt your head from side to side, forward, and backward to stretch the neck muscles.
- Rotate your head to either side.
- These stretches aid in decreasing neck tension and preserving neck mobility.

Always visit a healthcare practitioner or physical therapist before beginning a new fitness routine, particularly if you have existing spinal issues or concerns. They may give coaching on routines targeted to your demands and constraints. Remember to start lightly, keep optimal form, and gradually raise the intensity to save your spine and boost its health.

Preventive Measures for High-Risk Groups

Preventive measures for high-risk populations to minimize the probability of acquiring a neck hump (kyphosis) or to regulate its development include:

1. **Maintain Good Posture:**
   - High-risk groups, such as those with a family history of kyphosis or those who participate in activities that place additional pressure on the spine, should be especially sensitive to their posture. Avoid slouching, rounding the shoulders, and retaining a forward head position.
2. **Regular Exercise:**
   - Engage in exercises that concentrate on strengthening the muscles that support the spine, specifically the back and core muscles. This helps retain proper posture and spinal alignment. Incorporate workouts like yoga, Pilates, and strength training into your program.
3. **Ergonomics:**
   - If you have an employment that entails extended sitting, ensure sure your workplace is ergonomically structured. Use seats and workstations that offer appropriate lumbar support and encourage good posture.
4. **Backpack Safety:**
   - High school and college students should pay attention to backpack safety. Ensure that the backpack is worn correctly, dispersing weight equally over both shoulders. Limit the weight of the backpack to avoid stress on the spine.

5. **Frequent Check-Ups:**
   - If you have a family history of kyphosis or other spinal diseases, consider frequent check-ups with a healthcare professional or orthopedic specialist. Early identification and intervention may help correct any spinal problems.

6. **Healthy Nutrition:**
   - Ensure that you maintain a balanced diet with a sufficient number of nutrients, mainly calcium and vitamin D, to promote bone health and growth.

7. **Postural Exercises:**
   - Incorporate specialized postural exercises into your program to maintain good posture and spinal health. These exercises may entail stretching and strengthening regimens focusing on the upper back, neck, and core muscles.

8. **Limit High-Impact Activities:**
   - If you are engaging in high-impact sports or activities that place considerable stress on the spine, consider decreasing your engagement or wearing suitable protective gear.

9. **Quit Smoking:**
   - If you smoke, consider ceasing. Smoking may substantially impact bone health and may lead to spinal diseases.

10.   **Stay Informed:**

- Educate yourself on the risk factors, symptoms, and early signs of kyphosis. This vigilance could lead to timely action if you see any substantial changes in your posture or spinal health.

CONCLUSION

In conclusion, this book has studied the wide world of the neck hump, casting light on its numerous features, from its causes and risk factors to its cure and prevention. Our trip through the pages has revealed the need to treat this condition, not just as a cosmetic concern but as a critical component of comprehensive health and well-being.

We have determined that kyphosis, or the neck hump, is not a discrete illness but rather a condition with different origins and characteristics. Its development is affected by both inherited and environmental variables, underscoring the necessity of early identification, quick treatment, and continuous care.

Through these pages, we have shown the vital role of posture in spine health, emphasizing that prevention remains the most effective weapon against the neck hump. Education, awareness, and preventive measures have been our allies in this effort, driving high-risk groups and people alike toward a healthier, more upright future.

This book has also investigated the different therapy choices available, demonstrating that although a comprehensive "cure" may not always be attainable, major improvements and symptom management are within reach. The significance of early intervention, individualized strategies, and multidisciplinary treatment has been consistently emphasized throughout these pages.

In the end, the quest to grasp and resolve the neck hump serves as a testament to the tenacity of the human spirit, the ability for healing, and the significance of knowledge. We want the knowledge and concepts offered within these pages to empower people to take charge of their spinal health, seek expert help when required, and live a life that stands tall in both body and spirit. As we continue our assessment, may the route to spinal health and well-being be created with knowledge, dedication, and the unshakable confidence that a life free from the obligations of the neck hump is well within reach.